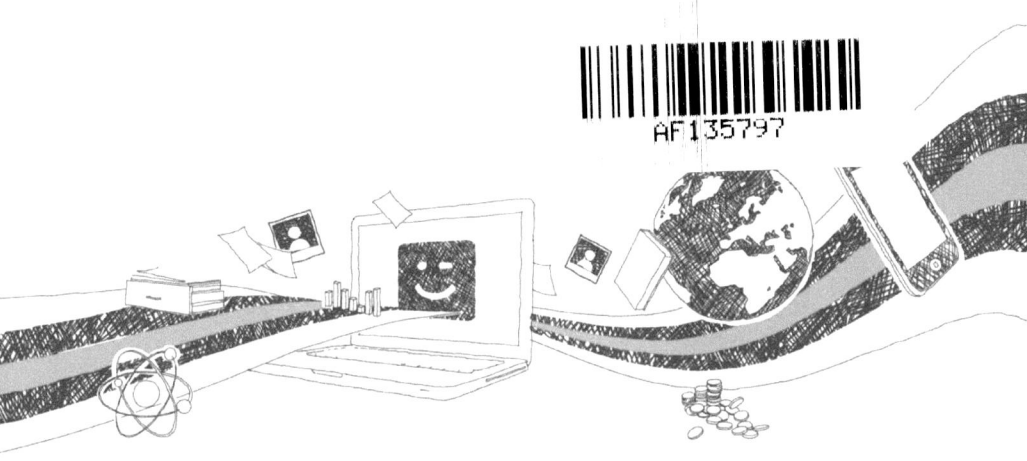
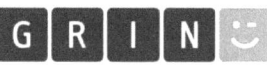

Bibliographic information published by the German National Library:

The German National Library lists this publication in the National Bibliography; detailed bibliographic data are available on the Internet at http://dnb.dnb.de .

Imprint:

Copyright © 2018 GRIN Verlag
Print and binding: Books on Demand GmbH, Norderstedt Germany
ISBN: 9783346025579

This book at GRIN:

https://www.grin.com/document/497956

Katja Grasberger

A cross-cultural comparison of Patient-Centered Communication and empathy on Ask-The-Expert healthcare websites

GRIN Verlag

GRIN - Your knowledge has value

Since its foundation in 1998, GRIN has specialized in publishing academic texts by students, college teachers and other academics as e-book and printed book. The website www.grin.com is an ideal platform for presenting term papers, final papers, scientific essays, dissertations and specialist books.

Visit us on the internet:

http://www.grin.com/

http://www.facebook.com/grincom

http://www.twitter.com/grin_com

RHEINISCHE FRIEDRICH-WILHELMS-UNIVERSITÄT BONN

Institut für Anglistik, Amerikanistik und Keltologie

"Weiter so! - There is light at the end of the tunnel!"

A Cross-Cultural Comparison of Patient-Centered Communication and Empathy

on Ask-The-Expert Healthcare Websites

Katja Grasberger

Table of contents

1. Introduction

The evolution of the internet permanently offers its users new possibilities and opportunities to have access to a variety of services at the comfort of the own home. Ask-the-expert advice-giving websites and forums have become common in the world wide web, to provide users with lay person or expert opinions and support on specific topics. Online health support and intervention has become particularly popular, is frequently used by the online community and indeed offers several advantages. By using online healthcare services, costs for health service are reduced, the convenience for users is increased, the stigma for certain conditions is lowered and information is made readily available for users (cf. Griffiths et al. 2006). While it has been the quality and accuracy of internet health information that was investigated in medical research (e.g. Ademiluyi, Rees and Sheard 2003), the interactive and communicative functions have been rather neglected.

Next to interactive and communicative functions, the use of empathy and patient-centered communication (PCC) on online healthcare websites have also only been infrequently investigated. Studies (eg. Little et. al 2001, Bonvicini 2009) have provided evidence that the usage of empathy in clinical consultations can increase patient satisfaction, adherence to treatment plans and recovery rates. It is especially patients with psychosocial problems that have been found to be more likely to want and expect PCC (cf. Winefield 1995) in medical consultations. While it is widely accepted that empathy and PCC is key to successful medical face-to-face consultations (cf. Mead & Bower 2002), some research (e.g. Lovejoy et. al 2009) has suggested that emphatic communicative strategies are harder to achieve in online communication. It has even been suggested that empathy and PCC might not be deemed important by either the online expert and the patient (cf. Pounds 2016).

This study investigates whether online healthcare experts from Germany and the UK make use of empathy and PCC in their expert responses to online patients struggling with depression. The study primarily focuses on cross-cultural differences and similarities for which a discourse-analytical approach is used to analyze relevant communicative strategies. Based on the findings, the study aims to deduce possible implications and questions whether cultural awareness is needed in online ask-the-expert healthcare contexts. I claim that empathy and PCC is used differently in online healthcare context in Germany and the UK.

The paper starts with the theoretical background providing a comprehensive overview including general advice research, specifically on ask-the-expert online websites, in the light of empathy and PPC. The methodology chapter will present details of the data collected and the coding scheme used. The fourth chapter includes most important findings which are relevant to answer the research questions. The discussion chapter will be used to look at the results in the light of previous findings and theories. At last, the paper will close with a summary of all relevant and noteworthy findings and will offer an outlook and ideas for future research worth investigating to get greater insights.

2. Theoretical Background

Human beings ask and receive advice on a daily basis, whether it takes place in private or public sphere, face-to-face or even online. The online Merriam-Webster Dictionary defines *advice* as a "recommendation regarding a decision of course of conduct: counsel", the online Oxford Learner's Dictionary defines it as "an opinion or a suggestion about what somebody should do in a particular situation" and the online Collins Dictionary as a "recommendation as to a appropriate choice of action; counsel". All definitions describe scenarios in which advice-givers give their opinion, suggestion or recommendation on how to solve a problem. It implies that if the advice-receiver implements the given recommendations, it will be beneficial for him or her. The act of advising is, however, in itself critical. While it has been found that in some cultures, such as Japanese, Korean or Chinese, to give advice can be a sign of solidarity, there are other cultures in which advice-giving is rather considered face-threatening as for example in Anglo-Western contexts (Locher 2006: 4). In contexts in which advice is perceived as threatening, Goldsmith and MacGeorge (2000: 235) claim that the hearer's identity as a competent social interlocutor is questioned. Locher (2006: 4) claims that thus a certain asymmetry between interactants exists which is perceived as threatening and may require mitigation such as praise or empathy. Another study by Morrow (2006) investigating advice on depression in an internet forum also reports that advice-givers make use of expressions with positive regard and solidarity. However, depression is a rather sensitive and delicate topic, which is why it is questionable whether it is the advice that attracts solidarity or the topic itself.

Bromme et al. (2005: 570) further examine advice from a communicative angle in online healthcare advice contexts stating that "online advice is a communicative activity that is demanding for both those who provide information and for those who request it". The essence of their definition is the joint activity of advice. Bromme et al. (2005: 570) suggest that it is already difficult in face-to-face interactions to establish a common ground between health experts and laypersons. Studies (e.g. Hall, Roter & Katz 1988) have shown that clinical experts talk more compared to their patients, but still must be careful not to overload the patient with expert terminology which would disturb the interaction if the patient does not understand what the expert is trying to say. If this is the case, the advice would eventually come to nothing and would not be effective. Hence, it is important that both interlocutors take care of what the other is saying and adapt it to the respective context.

One such context to ask for and give advice are ask-the-expert healthcare websites. On ask-the-expert healthcare websites users have the opportunity to get informed about medical conditions and healthcare problems, but can also send in their own questions anonymously and ask for advice. The questions are then asynchronously answered by healthcare experts and are usually made public. The purpose of this is twofold: on the one hand this kind of communication serves a personal exchange, but at the same time serves the public as well (cf. Locher 2010: 48). Some other users of the website might identify with the same problem and find first points of advice. As mentioned above, while it is already challenging to find common ground in face-to-face interactions between experts and laypersons, computer-mediated communication obviously does not make it any easier. It is essential that healthcare experts linguistically adapt to their target audience. In the investigation of an American online healthcare advice service, *Lucy Answers*, Locher (2010: 55) has found that there is a general avoidance of technical vocabulary, except if the interlocutors asking for advice use it themselves. Humor and empathy are also readily used to create solidarity (cf. Locher 2010: 55). The interactive nature of virtual healthcare consultations have been investigated in a review by Dedding et al. (2011). Some of the disadvantages in online healthcare consultations listed are for example that patients cannot be directly investigated and that certain treatment plans cannot be translated into e-versions (cf. Dedding et al. 2011: 50). There are however also advantages for online patients, which can create improvements for patient participation. Due to the fact that online patients can anonymously ask for advice, they may, for instance, overcome stigmata for certain conditions and increase self-disclosure (cf. Dedding et al. 2011: 50-51). The review further reports a lever effect of online healthcare websites which may stimulate a changing process towards a more patient-centered care. However, the review does not offer any empirical evidence for the findings and the analyzed articles report rather contradictory effects on the patient-expert relationship in healthcare. Moreover, the studies included in the review mainly focus on situations in which a

3

patient-expert relationship already exists throughout previous face-to-face consultations. Pounds (2016: 119) claims that asynchronous exchanges with unknown experts "may be expected to be less conducive to the establishment of interpersonal rapport". Thus, Pounds (2016: 119) suggests that in these contexts patient-centeredness and mitigation strategies such as empathy might not be deemed as important by either interactant.

Nevertheless, patient-centered communication is a key feature in primary face-to-face healthcare interactions and is highly advocated (cf. Mead & Bower 2002). Stewart (2001: 445) states that "being patient centred [...] means taking into account the patient's desire for information and for sharing decision making and responding appropriately". This means that the patient and his or her needs take central stage and that the doctor must be considerate to give advice which is appropriate for the individual patient. Thus, PCC includes that the doctor has to be emphatic towards the patient on the one hand, but also involve him or her into future decisions and choices. Little et al. (2001: 1) elaborate on these characteristics by promoting five principles of a patient-centered model:

> exploring the experience and expectations of disease and illness, understanding the whole person, finding common ground regarding management (partnership), health promotion, and enhancing the doctor-patient relationship.

Patient-centeredness can have major benefits for patients. Little et al. (2001: 1) suggest that if it is applied correctly it can improve the patient's satisfaction and the medical development and recovery. Patient-centeredness is explicitly taught to physicians throughout their education, and studies (e.g. Little et al. 2001: 3–5) have shown that patients want and expect patient-centered communication when talking to their doctor. However, if patient-centeredness actually is exercised, it is restricted to individual characteristics of the doctor and the patient. A further question that arises is if the model provided by Little et al. (2001) can or should be implemented for all domains of healthcare practices. A cancer patient might need a different level of patient-centeredness compared to a patient with a foot placed in a plaster cast. It might really be dependent on the healthcare issue or problem itself that differences in preferences to patient-centeredness arise (cf. Little et al. 2001: 2). Supporting this, a study by Winefield (1995) has shown that it is especially patients with psychosocial problems that are more likely to want and expect a patient-centered consultation. The same study also shown that the doctor's patient-centeredness was highest for psychosocial consultations compared to complex and straightforward consultations (cf. Winefield 1995: 406). Conducting a literature review on patient-centeredness, Mead and Bower (2002) report several shortcomings of studies on patient-centeredness lacking high scores of internal and external validity. They claim that the typical investigated patient participant in their analyzed studies are female, mid-40 and married, which results in rather unvaried and unrepresentative outcomes (cf. Mead & Bower 2002: 59).

As already mentioned above, directly linked to patient-centeredness is the concept of empathy. Doctors should not only be sensitive regarding patients with psychosocial or other problems, but also display emphatic behavior. Ilie and Metea (2015: 214) define empathy as "an emotional understanding of other people's behavior […]". Being emphatic means to mirror the psychological state of the interlocutor in which his or her perspective is granted and acknowledged (Ilie & Metea 2015: 217). In an investigation of the impact of empathy on patient encounters, Bonvicini et al. (2009: 4) declare that empathy is a core part and essential to quality medical care. They report a meta-analysis of medical interactions by Beck et al. (2002) that found that a doctor's application of empathy is connected to higher scores in patient satisfaction, adherence, comprehension as well as to the perception of a good patient-expert relationship (cf. Bonvicini 2009: 4). In face-to-face patient-expert interactions, the expert is able to directly read the patient's gestures and body language which is crucial for communicating empathy or concern. In asynchronous computer-mediated communication this is not possible and has to be linguistically offset. Some researchers (e.g. Lovejoy et al. 2009) have suggested that PCC and emphatic communication is harder to realize in online communication. However, in her study on patient-centeredness and empathy on ask-the-expert healthcare website, Pounds (2016) has shown that experts from the UK make wide use of patient-centered and emphatic expressions in their online responses. All previously described restrictions do not hinder them to express their concern and sympathy with the online patient, although they have never met and most probably never will.

As mentioned earlier in this chapter, some studies (e.g. Locher 2006, Chentsova-Dutton & Vaughn 2012) have suggested cross-cultural differences in general advice giving. Locher (2006) claims that while in East Asian cultures advice-giving is perceived as welcome and a sign of solidarity, it is perceived as face-threatening in Anglo-Western cultures. Mitigation measures are, hence, more likely to appear in the latter in order not to attack the interlocutor's face. Chentsova-Dutton and Vaughn (2012) have shown that Russians were less likely to modulate their advice-giving behavior and more likely to describe advice as characteristic for supportive relationships. These studies suggest that advice-giving is a culturally dependent behavior and is realized and anticipated differently in different cultures. In the context of online ask-the-expert healthcare websites, research is rather scarce, with a few exceptions (e.g. Morrow 2006, Pounds 2018). Especially the investigation of PCC and empathy has so far exclusively been discussed by Pounds (2016) and Pounds and De Pablos-Ortega (2016). Although some medical studies (e.g. Saha et al. 2008) have emphasized the importance of both PCC and cross-cultural awareness in healthcare settings, there is, as to the knowledge of the author, only one systematic study by Pounds and De Pablos-Ortega (2016) which is concerned with the implementation of PCC and empathy in online ask-the-expert healthcare cross-cultural contexts. In this study, Pounds and De Pablos-Ortega (2016) report differences in expert responses on healthcare websites in the UK, Spain and Italy. While all experts make use of advice in their responses, Italian experts encourage self-disclosure, Spanish experts specifically focus on giving explanations and UK experts focus on advice, explanation and support (Pounds & De Pablos-Ortega 2016: 238). It is questionable, however, whether the study's results are fully comparable, because the sample sizes are rather different and range from 10 to 30 queries sampled. This present study aims at trying to add to the current research by investigating two ask-the-expert healthcare websites from the UK and Germany: *NetDoctor* and *Lifeline*.

3. Methodology

3.1. Data

German and English expert responses from health service advice interactions were collected from the German website *Lifeline* and from the UK website *NetDoctor* (cf. Appendix 1). Two subsequent corpora were created, each containing 20 expert responses amounting to a total of 40 responses. The expert responses all relate to queries dealing with depression.

The German website *Lifeline* was chosen, because it a well established healthcare website which is managed by the publishing company Funke-Mediengruppe. It offers a range of healthcare advice in the form of articles and expert discussion forums. The website is run and supported by doctors and medical journalists which interview experts, evaluate studies and attend medical congresses on a regular basis. They emphasize that the website's aim is not to substitute an actual doctor's appointment, but rather aim at increasing the quality of doctor-patient relationship by offering information. *Lifeline's* health advice services are free of charge and users who have medical questions only have to register to post a question. All doctors and their credentials are listed in the impress of the website. User's questions and expert responses that were sampled for the purpose of this study were posted between 2011 and 2017.

The website *NetDoctor* was chosen for investigation, because it is UK's leading independent healthcare website offering users access to a variety of different health information. *NetDoctor* is run by the publishing division Hearst Magazine UK. The website's operators claim that their aim is to break down medical language barriers and not replace a face-to-face doctor's appointment, meaning to simplify medical information so that it is understandable for everyone. Users have access to articles on conditions, healthy eating, medicines and frequently asked questions (FAQs) on different topics. *NetDoctor* further offers to answer personal medical questions, but advise users to search the archive section first. The archive section contains over 6,000 user-expert interactions in which doctors answer queries handed in by users. All expert responses were taken from the FAQs archive section on depression. The website lists all interacting doctors and their credentials on the 'About NetDoctor' section. All queries that were sampled for the purpose of this study were posted in 2011.

The topic depression was chosen, because, as Pounds (2016: 120) claims, "the experts' interpersonal communication skills are, arguably, particularly relevant in this context". Symptoms for depression cause suffering and interfere with a human's personal, social, work life and other important areas in a clinical meaningful way (cf. American Psychiatric Association 2013). Psychological strain is high for affected patients which is why medical advice should be especially patient-centered and emphatic.

3.2. Data Collection Procedure

Both questions and answers were collected in order to be able to look at each exchange as a whole. The answers were, hence, always analyzed in relation to the question posted. The expert responses all display responses to issues dealing with depression. The users in the forum were rather explicit about their problems, which could be due to the fact that the topic of depression itself has strong effects on human's emotions and actions. To answer the research questions of this study, only the answers to the queries were analyzed and coded.

Both websites offer specific platforms in which (non-)members can read and have access to queries posted by users. For this, *Lifeline* offers several publicly available discussion forums to which users can contribute for free. In the 'Expertenrat' forums, all queries are answered by qualified doctors. Posts from the individual 'Expertenrat' forum for depression were randomly sampled for the purpose of this study. The posts were either answered by individual doctors or by the 'Lifeline Gesundheitsteam' (cf. table 1). The 'Expertenrat' forum further offers the opportunity for users to reply to the doctor's response. Subsequent responses were by users, however, not collected.

Table 1. *Distribution of Expert Responses, German corpus*

Experts	German Corpus
Medical Team	16
Doctor A	1
Doctor B	3

Different to *Lifeline, NetDoctor* offers archives including several thousand queries and answers, which are made publicly available for (non-)members. Queries were either answered by one individual doctor, by two individual doctors or by the 'NetDoctor Medical Team' (cf. table 2). All expert responses were randomly sampled from the archive section on depression. If more than one doctor answered the same question, the expert responses were coded and analyzed as one.

Table 2. *Distribution of Expert Responses, UK corpus*

Experts	UK Corpus
Individual doctor A	8
A + B	8
NetDoctor Medical Team	4

Creating and using small-sized corpora has several advantages and disadvantages. Due to the small size of the corpora, all entries were manually sifted. This is on the one hand time-consuming and labour-intensive, but also offers the possibility to comprehensively analyze

8

qualitative data. Small corpora, however, also entail that only a small glimpse at linguistic phenomena is offered which hardly allows for a broader transfer onto a whole population. Despite its disadvantages, this method enables the researcher to look at each utterance individually in its own context. The researcher is therefore able to not only read what informants wrote, but also gets closer to what they actually mean. Hence, it must be noted that corpora only show its own contents and nothing more, meaning that generalizations "have to be treated as deductions, not as facts" (Hunston 2002: 23).

3.3. Coding Scheme

The coding scheme used for the analysis of the data is based on Pounds' (2016) theory- and corpus-driven analytical framework, which focuses on PCC and empathy in online ask-the-expert exchanges. Table 3 lists all codes and respective examples from the German and UK corpora. Letters and numbers in brackets after the examples indicate expert-response IDs. The German corpus is abbreviated with *GER* while the English corpus is abbreviated with *UK*. Examples from the German corpus were translated below the original examples. Both corpora were manually sifted and each occurrence was analyzed and coded in context to the initial query.

Table 3. *Overview of codes used to analyze expert responses*

Code	Examples
Empathy	
I. Eliciting Responding	*Are you depressed at the moment, do you think? (UK8)*
II. Acknowledging feelings	*It must feel like your worst nightmare. (UK10)*
III. Endorsing views	*Parallel ist […] eine Untersuchung sicher richtig und sinnvoll. (GER9)*
	(Translation: In parallel, an examination does certainly make sense.)
IV. Reference to details	*Sie studieren und machen keine einfache Ausbildung […] (GER19)*
	(Translation: You are studying and are not going through an easy education.)
V. Accepting	

- Positive judgement

Schön, dass Sie sich selbst schon auf dem Weg der Besserung sehen. (GER11)

(Translation: Great that you are already on the road to recovery.)

- Unconditional support

Hundreds of people report to GP surgeries with these types of symptoms every day. (UK2)

- Rejecting negative self-judgement

So, be kind to yourself – and don't keep telling yourself that you should be 'getting over it' yet. (UK1)

- Expression of encouragement

But there is light at the end of the tunnel. (UK2)

Sympathy

Wir hoffen, wir konnten Ihnen weiterhelfen (GER9)

(Translation: We hope we could offer help.)

Negative Empathy

I. Dismissing feelings

Please don't get too upset about this. (UK15)

II. Rejecting views

[...] I'm not convinced your man is trying to do that. (UK3)

III. Negative judgement

Denn letztendlich haben Sie sich auch ein Stück weit selbst dort hineinmanövriert.(GER18)

(Translation: In the end, you have partially maneuvered yourself into this situation.)

Advice

I. Explicit

- Open

[...] do try to talk to her about your feelings (UK4)

- Closed

Discuss your feelings with your GP. (UK1)

II. Implicit

Der entsprechende Spezialist bei solchen Erkrankungen ist der Facharzt für Psychosomatik oder Psychiatrie. (GER16)

(Translation: The respective specialist for such diseases is a psychosomatic consultant or psychiatrist.)

Explanation

Eine depressive Episode dauert im Durchschnitt 6 Monate (GER14)

(Translation: A depressive episode lasts 6 months on an average.)

As already defined above, it is widely agreed that empathy is a key feature to PCC (e.g. Bonvicini et al. 2009). This means that the doctor is able to understand patients, acknowledge their feelings and also include them in future choices and decisions. This can either be explicitly or implicitly communicated on ask-the-expert healthcare websites. These strategies are all listed below EMPATHY (I.—V.) in table 3 above. Studies have found that by expressing understanding and acknowledgement of another person's situations, people tend to use similar lexical or syntactical structures (e.g. Garrod & Pickering 2004). It has been suggested that implicit acknowledgement can also be achieved by orienting to other people's narrative through repetition or back-channelling (cf. Pounds 2016: 123). In a medical setting, doctors can use these mechanisms to signal that they are listening and understanding the problem. These kinds of communicative strategies are coded as empathy, as listed above.

The code SYMPATHY does not belong to empathy as it only conveys the speaker's but does not refer to the patient's feelings. It does still play an interactive role and has a patient-centered function (cf. Pounds & De Pablos-Ortega 2016)

A lack of empathy was coded as NEGATIVE EMPATHY and is defined as "showing lack of concern for the patient's perspective" (Pounds & De Pablos-Ortega 2016: 231). These denote expressions which include a dismissal or rejection of patients' feelings and also negative judgements about patients.

As clarified above, one of the characteristics of PCC is that the doctor involves the patient in future decisions and choices regarding medical treatment. Rather than directing the patient to start a specific treatment, the doctor can opt to give ADVICE to the patient. In the present study this was either explicitly or implicitly achieved. Explicit formulations were either coded as open, i.e. leaving options, or closed, i.e. leaving no options. Carefully giving advice and leaving the patient options is a balancing act for doctors and putting the patient at the center is essential.

The code EXPLANATION was used for occurrences in which doctors gave extra information on certain conditions and illnesses as well as on course of actions. The code OTHER was only used for occurrences which could not be sorted into any of the other categories.

Regarding the research questions, the main focus lies on the use of EMPATHY, NEGATIVE EMPATHY AND ADVICE. These three codes consist of empathy and PCC, or the lack of it, and show in how far doctors make use of empathic communicative strategies to convey PCC.

A discourse-analytical approach was used which means that speech acts are seen as single units of analysis with individual interactive functions within a wider speech event (cf. Pounds 2016). The occurrences in the expert responses were coded corresponding to core statements.

Hence, all expert responses contain several codes which stand next to each other, as in the following example:

(1) UK6: *I am so sorry that this is happening* [SYMPATHY] *but with good, prompt treatment the chances are that your partner will improve shortly.* [ACCEPTING: EXPRESSION OF ENCOURAGEMENT]

Although, in most cases one sentence was classified with one code, there were a few instances in which one sentence was given two codes as it represented more than one communicative function. The example below shows such a case where the utterance was coded as EMPATHY: ENDORSING VIEWS and ADVICE:EXPLICIT-OPEN.

(2) GER9: *Das Muttermal kann der Frauenarzt sicherlich zunächst auch begutachten, sollte aber bei Unklarheiten dermatologisch gesehen werden.*

(Translation: The birthmark can certainly first be assessed by a gynecologist, but should be dermatologically tested in case of unclarity.)

On first sight, the example above might only be coded as an ADVICE. The initial question however already includes the user's thoughts on going to see her gynecologist, which makes example 2 also an emphatic expression endorsing the user's views. These cases occurred only occasionally and marked exceptions.

Some codes consist of rather long sentences, while others only include short phrases. It was sometimes difficult to define the starting and ending point of a code, and when in doubt the whole sentence was coded. Eventually, 98% of the sentences and phrases produced by the experts could be sorted into one of the predefined codes by Pounds (2016) and no additional code had to be added.

4. Results

4.1. Realization of PPC and Empathy

In both, the German and English corpora, the online patients exploit the medium to disclose their feelings and problems to seek medical or rather psychological help and advice. However, German online patients use more words in their queries than English online patients. On average, German queries amount to 303 words, while in the English corpus the queries consist of 183 words. This is also true for the overall word count. In the German corpus, queries make up 67 %, while in the English corpus queries make up only 37 %. This means that either German online patients use far more words than experts in their responses, or that German experts generally use less words compared to the English experts. The results show however that the latter is more likely: with an average of 310 words per response in the English corpus, experts from the UK use twice as much words compared to the German experts, which used 151 words on average in their responses. The average of one exchange are however quite similar for both corpora and amount to 453 words per exchange in the German corpus and to 492 words per exchange in the English corpus. This provides evidence for the picture that German experts respond with less words compared to the English experts. Nevertheless, this should not be mistaken as an assumption that German experts are less patient-centered or use less empathy in their responses than English experts just because the word count in different in comparison.

An overview of both the German and English results is displayed in table 4 and table 5 respectively below. Both tables list all categories with their total and relational occurrences. Percentages are used throughout the following tables and figures due to the fact that occurrences found in each corpus highly varied, which is why it makes more sense to report strategies by the size of their shares to overall occurrences of the respective corpus.

The overall results showed that the German expert responses included 196 occurrences, while the English expert responses included 282 occurrences which all served a communicative function. The German corpus amounted to a word count of 9,065 words, while the English corpus consisted of 9,846 words (both queries and responses were counted). Expert responses from the German website *Lifeline* consist of less words and communicative strategies compared to the English website *NetDoctor*. This implies that on the German website online patients make use of a lot of words to describe their feelings, and experts give rather short answers compared to the English website for which it is the other way around.

Table 4. *Overview of results: German data*
Total Number of Words in Corpus: 9,065

	Category (Pounds 2018)	Occurrences	%
EMPATHY	Eliciting Responding	9	4.6 %
	Acknowledging feelings	9	4.6 %
	Endorsing views	8	4.1 %
	Reference to details	6	3.1 %
	Accepting (total)	**30**	**15.3 %**
	Positive judgement	3	1.5 %
	Unconditional support	10	5.1 %
	Rejecting negative self-judgement	5	2.6 %
	Expression of encouragement	12	6.1 %
	TOTAL	**62**	**31.6 %**
	Sympathy	**28**	**14.3 %**
NEGATIVE EMPATHY	Dismissing feelings	0	0.0 %
	Rejecting views	2	1.0 %
	Negative judgement	10	5.1 %
	TOTAL	**12**	**6.1 %**
ADVICE	Explicit	25	12.8 %
	Open	19	9.7 %
	Closed	6	3.1 %
	Implicit	26	13.3 %
	TOTAL	**51**	**26.0 %**
	Explanation	**38**	**19.4 %**
	Other	**5**	**2.6 %**
	GRAND TOTAL	**196**	100.0 %

Table 5. *Overview of results: UK data*

Total number of words in corpus: 9,846

	Category (Pounds 2018)	Occurrences	%
EMPATHY	Eliciting Responding	5	1.8 %
	Acknowledging feelings	21	7.4 %
	Endorsing views	7	2.5 %
	Reference to details	7	2.5 %
	Accepting (total)	**65**	**23.0 %**
	Positive judgement	14	5.0 %
	Unconditional support	17	6.0 %
	Rejecting negative self-judgement	4	1.4 %
	Expression of encouragement	30	10.6 %
	TOTAL	**105**	**37.2 %**
	Sympathy	**22**	**7.8 %**
NEGATIVE EMPATHY	Dismissing feelings	3	1.1 %
	Rejecting views	6	2.1 %
	Negative judgement	18	6.4 %
	TOTAL	**27**	**9.6 %**
ADVICE	Explicit	63	22.3 %
	Open	36	12.8 %
	Closed	27	9.6 %
	Implicit	32	11.3 %
	TOTAL	**95**	**33.7 %**
	Explanation	**30**	**10.6 %**
	Other	**3**	**1.1 %**
	GRAND TOTAL	**282**	100.0 %

As mentioned above the core categories most important for this study are ADVICE, EMPATHY and NEGATIVE EMPATHY. If it is true that German and English experts make use of PCC and empathy, numbers for EMPATHY and ADVICE should be high, while, logically, numbers for NEGATIVE EMPATHY should be low. Subcategories of EMPATHY all consist of communicative strategies which aim to give the patient the feeling of acknowledgment and acceptance, which are core characteristics of empathy and PCC. As described in chapter two, another characteristic of PCC includes the patient in future decisions on treatment and is represented as the code ADVICE in this present study.

Both German and English experts make vast use of empathy and PCC in their responses. ADVICE and EMPATHY are the most common categories found in both the German and the English corpus. In the German corpus, EMPATHY makes up 31.6 % (62 occurrences) of all expert responses while it amounts to 37.2 % (105 occurrences) in the English corpus. The category ADVICE was identified for 26.0 % (51 occurrences) of cases in the German corpus, while it appeared in 33.7 % (95 occurrences) of the cases in the English corpus. NEGATIVE EMPATHY was the least favorite strategy for German experts (6.1 %, 12 occurrences) and was also the least popular strategy among English experts (9.6 %, 27 occurrences). Although there are some instances of negative empathy, the use of empathy and PCC prevailed and was much higher.

The results provide evidence that both English and German experts apply PCC and empathy in online healthcare consultations. Experts from both websites seem to focus first on empathy and secondly on solution-oriented advice. While both expert groups only rarely displayed negative empathy English experts made more use of it than German experts. Nevertheless, NEGATIVE EMPATHY was far less used compared to EMPATHY and ADVICE which implies that empathy and PCC is an important tool which is commonly used among online healthcare experts.

4.2. Cross-cultural comparison

The previous chapter has dealt with the first research question, whether English and German experts make use of empathy and PCC in online healthcare consultations. This chapter will deal with the second research question and investigates in how far English and German experts use empathy and PCC differently or similarly in terms of categories used. An overview of the core categories is presented in figure 1 below.

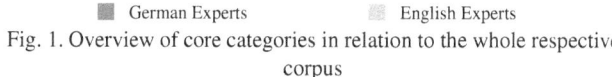

German Experts   English Experts

Fig. 1. Overview of core categories in relation to the whole respective corpus

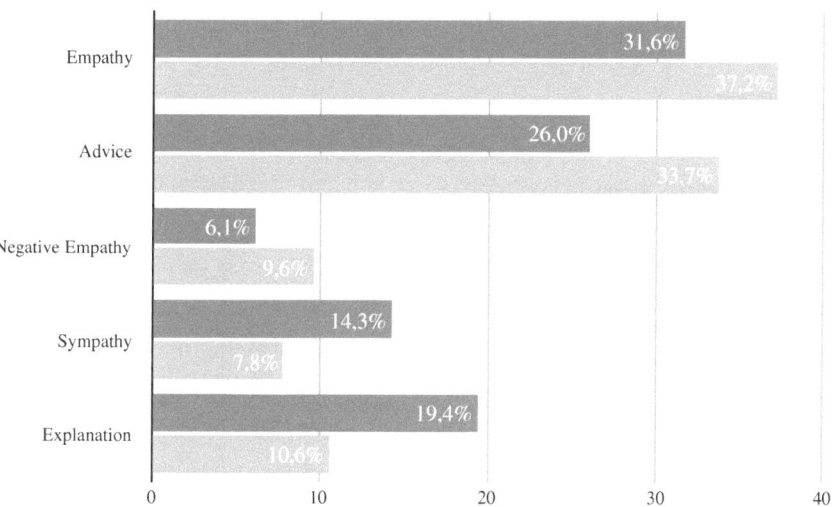

As already mentioned in the previous chapter, the categories EMPATHY and ADVICE are most frequently used in online expert consultations which speaks for an extensive use for PCC and empathy. NEGATIVE EMPATHY was used by both German and English experts, but was generally lower compared to strategies connected to empathy and PCC. The usage of SYMPATHY and EXPLANATION is not the main focus of this paper as it is not directly linked to empathy, but will shortly be commented on. German experts used far more sympathetic strategies compared to English experts, and also made more use of medical explanations. The use of sympathy appeared to have a rather conventional form and almost exclusively appeared at the end of the response in the German corpus and was realized as *Wir hoffen wir konnten Ihnen weiterhelfen* (Translation: We hope we could help.) in over 50 % of the responses. No such favored placement was found in the English responses. Both German and English experts use explanations most commonly right after ADIVE or EMPATHY STRATEGIES, as demonstrated in example 3 below.

(3) UK2: *Hundreds of people report to GP surgeries with these types of symptoms every day.*
[ACCEPTING: UNCONDITIONAL SUPPORT] *You are certainly not alone and the good
news is that help is available.* [ACCEPTING: EXPRESSION OF ENCOURAGEMENT]

*Your physical symptoms of headaches, fatigue, insomnia and appetite fluctuations are
classically seen in these type of problems.* [EXPLANATION]

It is not surprising that doctors might use these combinations, as explanations may serve doctors
to demonstrate knowledge to justify their advice or to make patients feel better in combination
with empathy.

Realizing positive EMPATHY is most commonly realized in the form of acceptance on
both healthcare websites, amounting to 23.0 % (65 occurrences) in the English responses and
15.3 % (30 occurrences) in the German responses. Both use EXPRESSION OF
ENCOURAGEMENT most frequently, in 10.6 % (30 occurrences) of the cases in the English
corpus and 6.1 % (12 occurrences) in the German corpus. The second most popular subcategory
of ACCEPTING was UNCONDITIONAL SUPPORT, again for both healthcare expert groups.
English experts further used POSITIVE JUDGEMENTS (5.0 %, 14 occurrences), while this
category was the least favorite among German experts in the ACCEPTING category (1.5 %, 3
occurrences). ACCEPTING makes up around 50 % of empathy strategies in both corpora.

Looking at the other empathy strategies outside of acceptance, some similarities and
differences can be found as well. The most frequent strategy there was ACKNOWLEDGING
FEELINGS with 7.4 % (21 occurrences) in the English corpus and 4.6 % (9 occurrences) in the
German corpus. The strategy ELICITING RESPONDING was further used by German experts
as frequently as ACKNOWLEDGING FEELINGS which is different to the English corpus in
which this category is the least frequent. This might be due to the fact that on the German
website it is actually possible for online patients to respond to the expert's response, while this is
not possible on the English website. German online doctors might, thus, make more use of
strategy ELICITING RESPONDING, because patients are able to answer. However, the use of
ELICITING FEELINGS still occurred in some English responses, but seem to be rather used as
food for thought and kind of have a preparatory function as in the following example:

(4) UK13: *Why is it so difficult for you, do you think?* [ELICITING RESPONDING]
I'm not sure quite how long you've been taking your antidepressant (Seroxat) for?
[ELICITING RESPONDING]

It looks as though it is probably three months, or longer. But if it's not working, then you should ask the doctor to consider changing you to another one. [ADVICE: EXPLICIT-OPEN]

Both questions in this example do not require an answer to proceed in the interaction, but rather prepare the upcoming usage of ADVICE. This could be interpreted as a hedging tool, to lower the level of imposition of the upcoming advice.

ADVICE strategies were generally the second most frequent strategies used by both German (26.0 %, 51 occurrences) and English (33.7 %, 95 occurrences) experts. As already mentioned in the methodology chapter, advice was either realized implicitly or explicitly in closed (i.e. leaving no options) or open (i.e. leaving options) form, whereas implicit strategies are always open. Figure 2 gives an overview of these strategies.

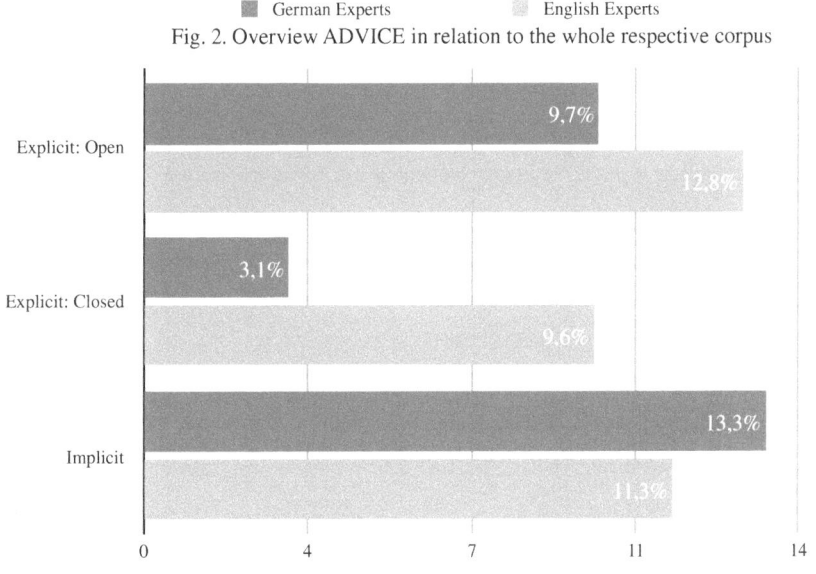

■ German Experts   English Experts
Fig. 2. Overview ADVICE in relation to the whole respective corpus

In the German corpus, explicit and implicit strategies balance each other while in the English corpus explicit advice is more common than implicit advice. If German and English experts used an explicit advice, it appeared more often in open form than in closed form. This means that although an explicit form was usually preferred by both expert groups, they still opted to keep the level of imposition as low as possible. Further, English experts seemed to be more comfortable using closed explicit advice strategies (9.6 %, 27 occurrences) compared to the German experts (3.1 %, 6 occurrences).

Expressions of NEGATIVE EMPATHY were uncommon in the collected expert responses and only made up 6.1 % (12 occurrences) in the German corpus and 9.6 % (27 occurrences) in the English corpus. The strategy NEGATIVE JUDGEMENT was least frequently used by both expert groups. The strategy DISMISSING FEELINGS was the only strategy that did not occur once in the German corpus and was also only scarcely used by English experts responses (1.1 %, 3 occurrences).

5. Discussion

The present paper investigated whether healthcare online experts from Germany and the UK, first of all, generally make use of empathy and PCC in their online healthcare expert responses and if so, how these cultural groups differ or are similar in terms of communicative strategies used to achieve the former. The limited amount of data offers just a glimpse into how empathy and PCC can be realized in an online healthcare consultation setting and does not allow for general conclusions. Nevertheless, the results presented in this paper allowed for a small overview of how German and English healthcare experts use emphatic communicative strategies to respond to online patients suffering from depression.

The overall results show that both German and English experts make use of PCC and empathy in their responses to online patients. Word frequencies presented indicated that German online patients used more words to describe their condition than experts used to realize their response, while it was the other way around in the English corpus. However, previous studies (e.g. Hall, Roter and Katz 1988) have suggested that clinical experts generally speak more in face-to-face consultations than patients. Word frequencies in English expert responses would fit to this finding, but not the German expert responses. However, in their meta-analysis Hall, Roter and Katz (1988) do not specify any cultural settings in which their investigated studies took place, which is why comparability is rather questionable. Although German and English expert responses differ in word count, all include several occurrences of empathy and PCC strategies

(EMPATHY and ADVICE most prominently) to sensitively respond to their online patients. This is in line with previous findings provided by Pounds (2016) and Pounds and De Pablos Ortega (2016) which did not only analyze and found emphatic communicative strategies but also looked at cultural differences.

The results of the German and English expert responses displayed no big differences in terms of empathy and PCC used. The most frequent strategies used in the present study were EMPATHY and ADVICE in both German and English expert responses making up over 50 % of all strategies used in both corpora. When using emphatic strategies, both expert groups most frequently made use of ACCEPTING strategies to display support and encouragement. This is also in line with Pounds (2016) findings on the same matter. While emphatic strategies primarily display similarities between German and English experts, it is the use of ADVICE that shows some differences. Generally, German expert responses consisted of a balanced use of explicit and implicit strategies, although open explicit advice was more common than closed explicit advice. English expert responses on the other hand consisted of more explicit strategies than implicit strategies, but still slightly favored open explicit advice strategies. Studies have found (e.g. Locher 2006, Goldsmith & MacGeorge 2000) that advice may be perceived as face-threatening especially by Anglo-Western cultures and is thus most often mitigated to lower the level of imposition. The results of this study are consistent with this finding and suggest that although medical advice is actually asked for on this kind of websites, it is still realized in a mitigated and careful way. PCC seems to play a role and is important in this kind of interaction, as this kind of advice actually leaves patients options and involves them in future treatment and action. This kind of positive and solution-oriented communication seems to be especially important for psychosocial problems, which have been found to be characteristic in online healthcare advice interactions for depression in other studies (cf Morrow 2006). Nevertheless, it could also very well be that advice is realized in a more open way, because both websites claim not to offer any diagnoses. This may cause the realization of advice to be more indicative.

Additionally, the realization of EXPLANATIONs seems to be different as well. The results show that German experts used more explanations in addition to other strategies, compared to English experts. The explanations in both corpora are rather extensive and usually consisted of a row of clauses and sentences. Moreover, experts abstain from using too specific expert vocabulary, which highlights the interactional value of online healthcare communication. This is in line with previous findings (e.g. Locher 2010) claiming that experts try to elude technical vocabulary. It seems that on both German and English websites, experts try to adapt to the linguistic level of their online patient by not using too many technical terms. Interestingly, however, if English experts use technical terms *NetDoctor* directly provides a solution by hyperlinking specific terms to explanation websites. This is especially helpful as online patients do not get the chance to reply to the expert and ask further questions. Such hyperlinks are not offered on the German website *Lifeline*, but patients can actually reply to doctors if they want to and have further questions.

The case of NEGATIVE EMPATHY appeared to be not as straightforward as it seemed. All categories consisting of negative empathy were designed to mark occurrences where the opposite of empathy takes place. There are however not only occurrences of NEGATIVE EMPATHY where the doctor aims to be negatively judgmental, but also occurrences in which the lack of empathy actually seems to have an accepting, encouraging and acknowledging tone. The following examples from both corpora are instances where negative empathy may also be interpreted as emphatic.

(5) GER18: *Dass das Problem ganz wo anders liegt und es nicht nur "vielleicht" am Stress liegt, sondern Sie maximal ausgebrannt sind, dazu braucht es keinen Facharzt.* [NEGATIVE EMPATHY: NEGATIVE JUDGEMENT]

(Translation: That the problem lies somewhere else and it is not only "maybe" due to the stress, but you burned out to the maximum, does not need the judgement of a specialist.)

(6) UK3: *If he never meets you even halfway you'll go on feeling bleak and empty and there's only so much of that that anyone can take.* [NEGATIVE EMPATHY: NEGATIVE JUDGEMENT]

Both instances do not depict classic examples of negative judgement of the patient him or herself, but rather a negative judgement about the patient's negative judgement. This gives the negative judgement a tone of encouragement and empathy as it rejects the negative judgement of the patient. It would be interesting to investigate how patients perceive and would react to this ambiguity and whether it would cause misunderstandings.

With only 20 expert responses in each corpus, by far not all expert responses from these website were collected and there are many more websites offering the same service with different principles to reply to healthcare queries. Due to the fact that German online patients can actually reply to the expert responses, it might very well be that experts might produce their responses with this fact in their mind. If it is the case that patients have further questions, they can easily use the comment function below the expert response. On the English website, patients cannot as easily leave a comment to ask further questions. This might also be the reason why word count in German expert responses first of all are much lower than in the original queries and secondly also much lower compared to English expert responses. German experts have the chance to respond several times if it is necessary so there is no need to pack all the information into one response. Although the amount of data collected for this study is limited, it still offers a glimpse into how different cultural groups make use of empathy and PCC on healthcare websites, specifically in depression forums.

6. Conclusion

The main research questions of this study was first of all whether German and English experts from ask-the-expert healthcare websites make use of empathy and PCC in their responses to queries dealing with depression and secondly investigated cross-cultural differences in terms of communicative strategies used to achieve the former. By using a discourse-analytical approach, the present study provided a qualitative and quantitative analysis of expert responses from the German healthcare website *Lifeline* and the UK based healthcare website *NetDoctor* to answer both research questions. Although the results indicate no big difference in the use of empathy and PCC, it has been shown that online experts make use of a broad range of emphatic communicative strategies on ask-the-expert healthcare websites, to carefully and emphatically respond to queries and offer advice. Even if the amount of data is limited and does not allow for general conclusions, the results presented in this paper indicate several implications in terms of cross-cultural differences and similarities.

The findings of this study have shown that empathy and PCC is frequently used both in German and English expert responses. The core principles of PCC include that doctors are emphatic towards patients, but also involve them into future decisions and choices by offering advice in terms of treatment. In this study this was realized by EMPATHY and ADVICE strategies. If empathy and PCC is actually used in healthcare expert responses, values for EMPATHY and ADVICE should be high, while values for NEGATIVE EMPATHY should be low. It has been demonstrated that EMPATHY is the most frequently used strategy by both cultural expert groups which is predominantly realized as ACCEPTING. ADVICE strategies are the second most common strategies for both expert groups and included explicit and implicit advice strategies. The use of explicit and implicit strategies was balanced in German expert responses with a tendency to use more open explicit strategies than closed ones. Although English experts preferred to use more explicit advice strategies than implicit strategies, they also chose to use more open explicit advice strategies than closed ones.

NEGATIVE EMPATHY was the least popular strategy used for both cultural expert groups, while English experts made use of more such strategies than German experts. As already discussed, this category sometimes seemed to be inconclusive in terms of meaning. In some cases negative empathy was not used by the expert to really make, for example, a negative judgement with lack of empathy, but rather to reject negative judgements the patients made about themselves. In these cases, it could be argued that the negative judgement kind of serves as encouragement and support. It would be interesting to investigate how this is literally perceived by the patients.

The strategies SYMPATHY and EXPLANATION were not the main focus of this study, but were still coded as they are part of the expert responses. Sympathetic strategies and explanations were more frequently used by German experts than English experts. The use of sympathy usually appeared at the end of German expert responses. No such favored placement was found in the English expert responses. EXPLANATIONs most often appeared right after ADVICE and EMPATHY strategies. In this context, explanations might be used as a tool by the expert to justify advice or to make patients feel better by offering an explanation for their condition in combination with empathy.

Despite some limitations of the study at hand, the findings provide a documented overview of how online clinicians respond to queries dealing with depression. Manually analyzing each individual sample in connection to the original question posted is on the one hand surely time intensive, but also allows for a detailed qualitative analysis. All responses were analyzed in the context of the question posted which is important to understand the full meaning of each sentence. 20 expert responses for each cultural group is by far not enough to draw general conclusions and more extensive online ask-the-expert healthcare consultations must be analyzed to get greater insights. Nevertheless, findings of such studies can already raise an awareness that differences as well as similarities exist in terms of cultural values. It may enable experts to get insights in how their expressions are perceived in different cultural settings.

Further, it helps to analyze what patients of different cultural groups expect and receive online in comparison to face-to-face consultations.

More research needs to be done for other different cultural groups to find out about local and cultural practices and raise cultural awareness. The study presented here by no means includes all expert responses from each website and also might even missed out on other linguistic features that might have displayed bigger differences. This is no indicator that cultural awareness in this context is unneeded. Findings of such studies could help to build training material for doctors to bypass intercultural obstacles. Clinicians working in an international environment could then adapt their consultation style to offer the best medical consultation possible and not cause misunderstandings or frustration. It would also be interesting to investigate whether values for empathy and PCC are lower for somatic illnesses compared to psychosocial issues. It could be argued that the degree of suffering varies for different illnesses and that thus patients expect and experts offer a different kind of consultation style in an online setting. Finally, more research in this area may help to improve medical online as well as face-to-face consultations with clinicians, which ist especially relevant when it comes to intercultural overlaps.

References

Advice. (n.d.). In *Merriam-Webster online*. Retrieved August 15, 2018, from https://www.merriam-webster.com/dictionary/advice.

Advice. (n.d.). In *Oxford Learner's Dictionaries online*. Retrieved August 15, 2018, from https://www.oxfordlearnersdictionaries.com/definition/english/advice.

Advice. (n.d.). In *Collins Dictionary online*. Retrieved August 15, 2018, from https://www.collinsdictionary.com/dictionary/english/advice.

American Psychiatric Association. (2013). *Diagnostic and Statistical Manual of Mental Disorders* (5th ed.). Washington, DC: Author.

Ademiluyi, G., Rees, C., & Sheard, C. (2003). Evaluating the reliability and validity of three tools to assess the quality of health information on the Internet. *Patient Education And Counseling, 50*(2), 151–155.

Beck, Rainer S, Daughtridge, R. & Sloane, Philip D. (2002). Physician-patient communication in the primary care office: A systematic review. *The Journal of the American Board of Family Practice / American Board of Family Practice, 15*, 25–38.

Bonvicini, K., Perlin, M., Bylund, C., Carroll, G., Rouse, R., & Goldstein, M. (2009). Impact of communication training on physician expression of empathy in patient encounters. *Patient Education And Counseling, 75*(1), 3–10.

Bromme, R., Jucks, R., & Wagner, T. (2005). How to refer to 'diabetes'? Language in online health advice. *Applied Cognitive Psychology, 19*(5), 569–586.

Chentsova-Dutton, Y., & Vaughn, A. (2011). Let Me Tell You What to Do. *Journal Of Cross-Cultural Psychology, 43*(5), 687–703.

Dedding, C., van Doorn, R., Winkler, L., & Reis, R. (2011). How will e-health affect patient participation in the clinic? A review of e-health studies and the current evidence for changes in the relationship between medical professionals and patients. *Social Science & Medicine, 72*(1), 49–53.

Garrod, S., & Pickering, M. (2004). Why is conversation so easy?. *Trends In Cognitive Sciences*, *8*(1), 8–11.

Griffiths, F., Lindenmeyer, A., Powell, J., Lowe, P. and Thorogood, M. (2006). Why Are Healthcare Interventions Delivered Over the Internet? A Systematic Review of the Published Literature. *Journal of Medical Internet Research*, *8*(2), p.e10.

Goldsmith, D., & MacGeorge, E. (2000). The impact of politeness and relationship on perceived quality of advice about a problem. *Human Communication Research*, *26*(2), 234–263.

Hunston, S. (2002). *Corpora in Applied Linguistics*. Cambridge: Cambridge University Press.

Ilie, O., & Metea, I. (2015). Empathic And Assertive Communication. Efficient Communication Developments. *International Conference KNOWLEDGE-BASED ORGANIZATION*, *21*(1), 214–217.

Lifeline. Expertenrat Depressionen, Stress und Stressabbau. Retrieved August 15, 2018, from https://www.lifeline.de/expertenrat/leben-familie/depression-burnout-stress/.

Little, P. (2001). Preferences of patients for patient centred approach to consultation in primary care: observational study. *BMJ*, *322*(7284), 468–468.

Locher, M. (2006). *Advice online*. Philadelphia, PA: John Benjamins.

Locher, M. (2010). Health Internet sites: a linguistic perspective on health advice columns. *Social Semiotics*, *20*(1), 43–59.

Lovejoy, T., Demireva, P., Grayson, J., & McNamara, J. (2009). Advancing the practice of online psychotherapy: An application of Rogers' diffusion of innovations theory. *Psychotherapy: Theory, Research, Practice, Training*, *46*(1), 112–124.

NetDoctor. Depression - Ask the expert. Retrieved August 15, 2018, from https://www.netdoctor.co.uk/ask-the-expert/depression-faqs/.

Mead, N., & Bower, P. (2002). Patient-centred consultations and outcomes in primary care: a review of the literature. *Patient Education And Counseling*, *48*(1), 51–61.

Morrow, P. (2006). Telling about problems and giving advice in an Internet discussion forum: some discourse features. *Discourse Studies, 8*(4), 531–548.

Pounds, G. (2016). Patient-Centred Communication in Ask-the-Expert Healthcare Websites. *Applied Linguistics, 39*(2), 117–134.

Pounds, G., & De Pablos-Ortega, C. (2016). Patient-centred communication in British, Italian and Spanish 'Ask-the-Expert' healthcare websites. *Communication & Medicine, 12*(2–3), 225–241.

Hall, J., Roter, D., & Katz, N. (1988). Meta-analysis of Correlates of Provider Behavior in Medical Encounters. *Medical Care, 26*(7), 657–675.

Saha, S., Beach, M., & Cooper, L. (2008). Patient Centeredness, Cultural Competence and Healthcare Quality. *Journal Of The National Medical Association, 100*(11), 1275–1285.

Stewart, M. (2001). Towards a global definition of patient centred care. *BMJ, 322*(7284), 444–445.

Winefield, H., Murrell, T., Clifford, J., & Farmer, E. (1995). The usefulness of distinguishing different types of general practice consultation, or are needed skills always the same? *Family Practice, 12*(4), 402–407.

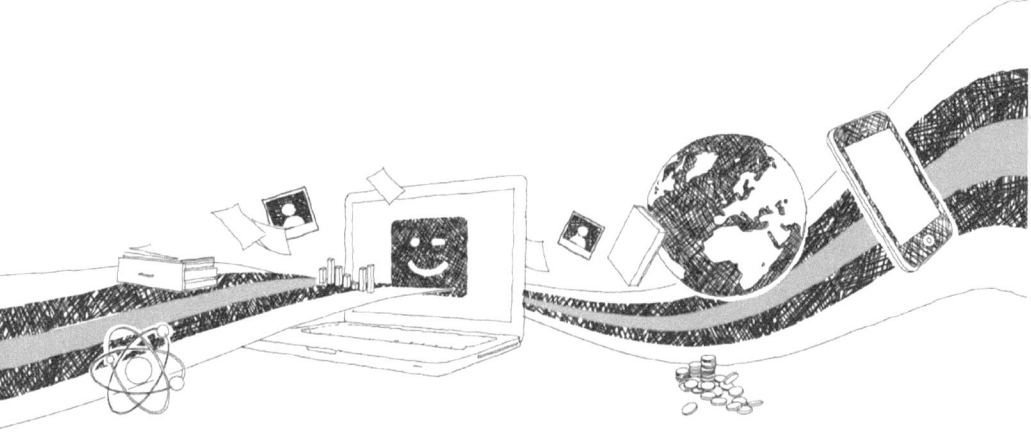